JOSE

I|

HEAD

GW00375233

JOSEPH CORVO'S INSTANT HEADACHE CURE

Joseph Corvo

CENTURY

LONDON SYDNEY AUCKLAND JOHANNESBURG

Published in 1991 by Century
Random Century Ltd
20 Vauxhall Bridge Road, London SW1V 2SA

Random Century Australia (Pty) Ltd
20 Alfred Street, Milsons Point, Sydney, NSW 2061, Australia

Random Century New Zealand Ltd
18 Poland Road, Glenfield, Auckland 10, New Zealand

Random Century South Africa (Pty) Ltd
PO Box 337, Bergvlei 2012, South Africa

Photographs © Barnaby Hopkins

Designed by Behram Kapadia
Set in Century Schoolbook and Univers
Printed and bound in UK by
Clays Limited, St Ives plc

A catalogue record for this book is available from the British Library.

ISBN 0-7126-5173-X

CONTENTS

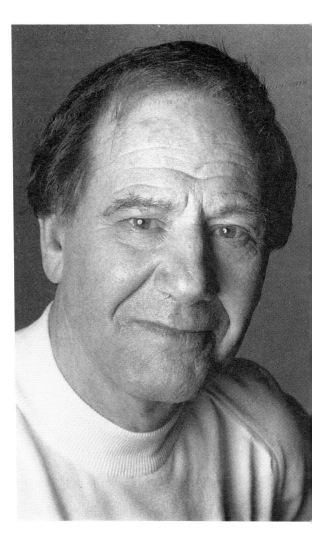

A MESSAGE FROM JOSEPH CORVO

The Zone Therapy revolution has begun. Until recently Zone Therapy was a secret I was able to share only with those relatively few people I could manage to treat personally, including members of the royal family and showbusiness celebrities. Following the publication of my first books, *Zone Therapy* and *The Natural Facelift*, the secret is out. Zone Therapy is now practised by millions of people all over the world. It has spread mainly by word of mouth *because it works*.

We all suffer from headaches now and then, many of us with a frequency that seriously disrupts our lives. The temptation is always to reach for pain-killing pills even though they are known to have damaging side-effects – after all, no drug is without them – and though the cost of these pills mounts up over the years.

Eliminating Pain

The good news is that there is another way. Zone Therapy is a system of pressure point massage which harnesses the body's own natural healing powers. By following the instructions contained in this book you can not only relieve the symptoms of headaches, migraines or hangovers in a way which is totally safe and free, but you can also heal whatever is causing this pain – and this is perhaps the most important difference between my headache cure and bottles of aspirin or paracetamol.

When you hurt yourself the natural impulse is always to rub it better. Zone Therapy enables you to direct this natural human impulse in a scientific manner. The results are miraculous.

Eliminating the Causes of Headaches

Headaches can have many different causes, nearly all of them to do with blockages in the body's nervous or electro-magnetic system which are in turn the result of a build-up of toxins in various key areas. These blockages are generally also aggravated by nervous tension – headaches are usually what we call distress signals.

More specifically the commonest causes of headaches are stress, neuralgia, inflamed sinuses, eye strain, tension in the back or neck, flu, earache, congestion of the sinus glands, over-indulgence in alcohol, and allergies. The programme that follows starts with a pressure point massage for relieving the pain, then proceeds with a systematic plan for finding and dealing with the range of possible causes by a process of elimination.

Follow the order I give you unless, of course, you have particular reason to believe you know the cause of your headache, in which case you must concentrate on the part of the programme which deals with that problem. For example, if you have a headache after having had too much to drink, it's likely that the cause of the pain will be a build-up of toxins in the liver; in this case working directly on the liver pressure point will achieve amazing results. If, on the other hand, you have been driving into the sun, the harsh glare may well have affected your eyes –

8

in which case work immediately on the pressure points for the eyes on your fingers.

Both the pain and the causes of most headaches can be eliminated by using the Instant Headache Cure on page 11. A persistent or recurring headache may need the more detailed programme on page 28.

If this treatment fails to eliminate a recurring head ache, you should see your doctor.

Joseph Corvo

THE INSTANT HEADACHE CURE
Joseph Corvo's 7 Point Plan

The aim of this 7 point, 7 minute programme is to eliminate both the pain and the cause of your headache.

So the next time you have a headache or migraine or hangover, instead of trying to numb the nerves with a pill, just push the pain out through the top of your head by following these instructions. It is surprisingly easy to do.

1 First, relieve the pain by pressing the roof of your mouth with your thumb, starting by pressing the middle of the roof of the mouth for thirty seconds, then pressing for thirty seconds on either side. Fourthly, press the roof of the mouth underneath the area of pain for the same length of time. For example, if the pain is around your left temple, press the area of the roof of the mouth directly behind the left canine tooth. If, on the other hand, the pain seems to be at the back of your skull, press the back of the roof of the mouth. If the pain seems to stem from the sinuses surrounding your right eye press the roof of the mouth at the front on the right.

2 Take the tips of the fingers of the left hand and press under the fingertips of the right hand. Put on as much pressure as you can for thirty seconds. Then take the tips of the fingers of the right hand and press under the

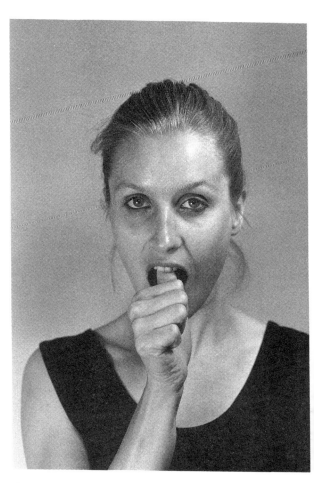

A quick and easy way of relieving pain.

fingertips of the left hand, also for thirty seconds.

Alternatively, if you have an aluminium comb, press it on to the fingertips as near to the fingernails (and thumbnails) as possible for thirty seconds on each hand.
3 The most direct approach to dealing with the sorts of tension and toxic build-up which cause headaches is by eliminating blockages in the pressure points on the hands.

Open the palm of your left hand to work on it with your right hand, using the thumb or first finger of your right hand to massage away the blockages which may have built up around the pressure points on your left hand.

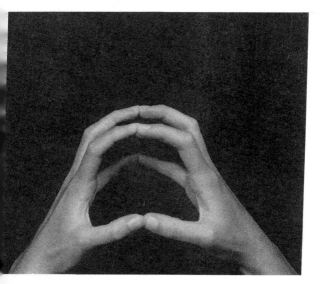

Pressing under fingertips of one hand with the nails of the other.

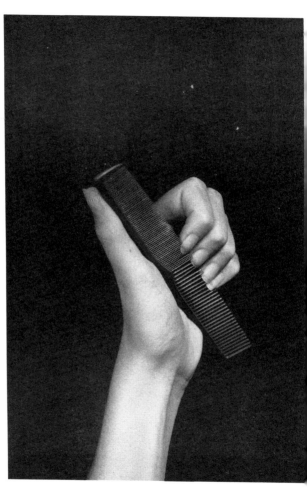

Pressing an aluminium comb under the fingertips.

Work on each pressure point for approximately twenty seconds, working as hard as you can with the thumb or forefinger rotating on a radius of half an inch. If a particular pressure point gives you pain, this is because it is congested; in which case continue working on it for another forty seconds.

Work on the pressure points in the following sequence:

(a) The brain

(b) The penial gland

(c) The pituitary gland

(d) The neck and
     cervicals

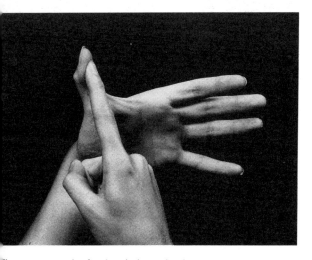

The pressure point for the pituitary gland.

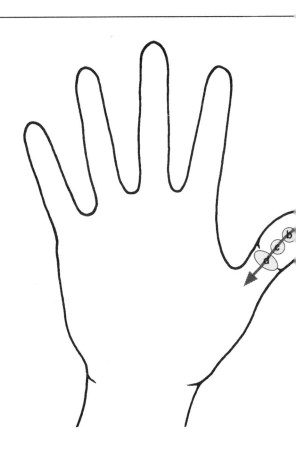

Working on the pressure points for the head: (a) the brain, (b) the penial gland, (c) the pituitary gland and (d) the neck and cervicals.

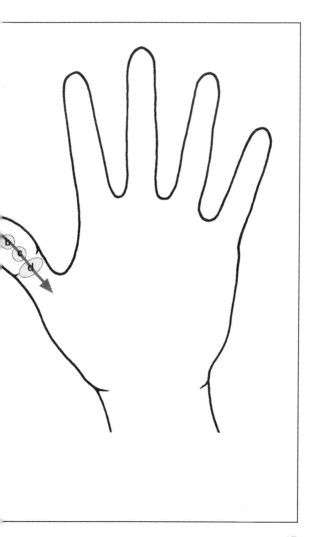

4 Then massage the pressure points for the ears, eyes and sinuses which run along the sides of the thumbs and fingers which face away from the body, and along the

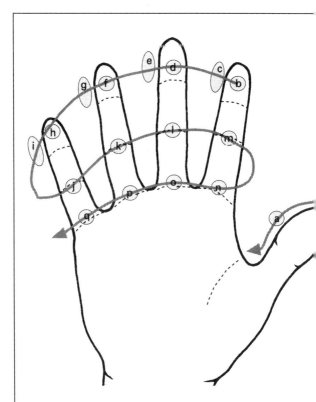

Working on the pressure points for the sinuses and also for the eyes and ears: points (j) to (m) and (n) to (q) run along the middle and bottom joints of the fingers.

joints of the thumbs and fingers. Inflamed or dehydrated sinuses are one of the commonest causes of headaches, as are eye strain and congestion of the ear:

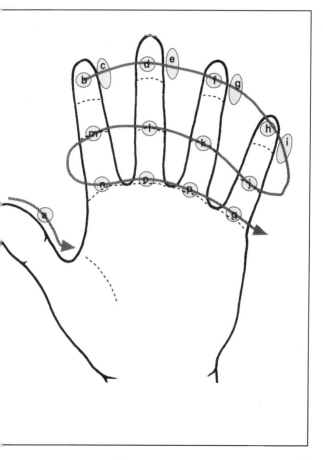

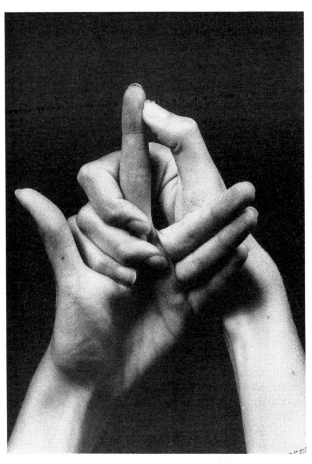

The pressure point for the eye sinus.

(a) Main sinus

(b) Eye

(c) Eye sinus

(d) Eye II

(e) Eye sinus II

(f) Ear

(g) Ear sinus

(h) Ear II

(i) Ear sinus II

(j) Ear Nerves

(k) Ear Nerves II

(l) Optical Nerve

(m) Optical Nerve II

(n) Eye III

(o) Eye IV

(p) Ear III

(q) Ear IV

5 Many headaches are caused by discomfort in the spine. Massage up and down the pressure points for the spinal column which run along the inside edge of the thumb down to the wrist; do this for thirty seconds on each hand.
6 Hangovers and other types of headaches are caused by a build-up of toxins in the liver. These can be reduced by working on the liver pressure point on the right hand as hard as you can for thirty seconds. (See p. 25)

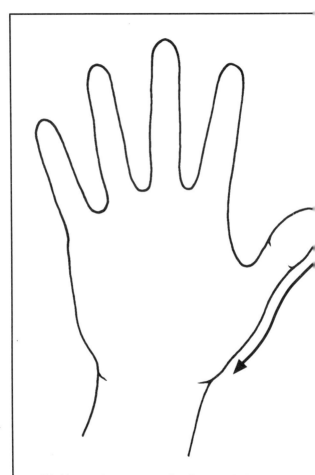

Working on the pressure points for the spinal column.

22

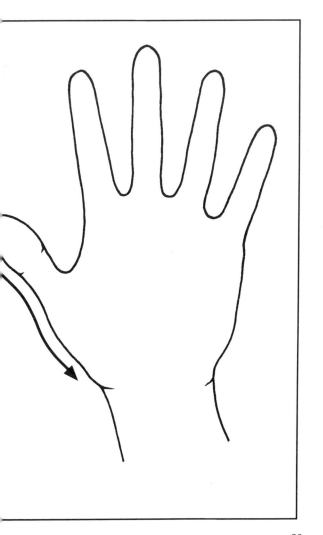

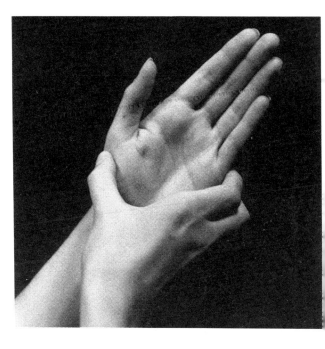

Working along the side of the hand to relieve tension in the back.

The pressure point for the liver.

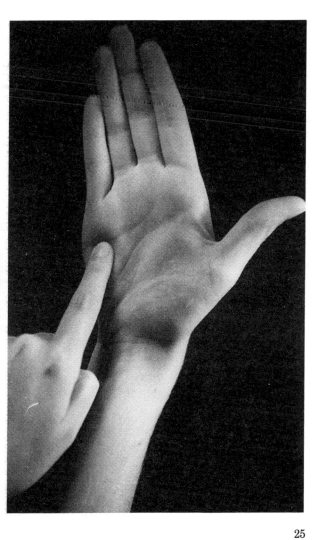

Another extremely effective way of eliminating toxins from the body is to massage the webbing between the thumb and the forefinger, stimulating the spot where the thumb and finger meet. Do this for one minute on each hand.

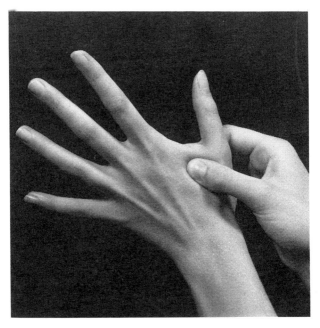

Working on the webbing between the thumb and forefinger.

7 Finally, massage the point where the back of the head joins the neck. Working this area will clear congestion of the lymph gland which is another common cause of headaches. Massage for one minute.

You will be amazed at the results.

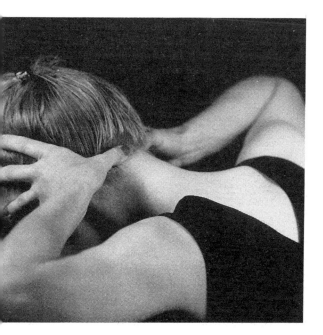

Working the point where the neck meets the head.

THE ZONE THERAPY CURE FOR PERSISTENT OR RECURRING HEADACHES

If this seven minute programme has not dealt with your headache, or if your headache regularly recurs, you may well have a more deap-seated problem, a more serious blockage somewhere in your system – and one serious blockage will tend to have a knock-on effect on related glands and nerves throughout your body. In this case I suggest you follow the forty-five minute programme detailed below. Forty-five minutes may seem a long time, but if you pursue this programme for just a few days, you can cure yourself of persistent headaches and also rid yourself of the other more serious problems which may be developing and of which your headaches may be just advanced symptoms. Again, if your headaches do not clear up you *must see a doctor*.

Start by relieving the pain by pressing the roof of your mouth with your thumb as hard as you can for thirty seconds on each of the following points:

1 The middle

2 The left

3 The right

4 Underneath the area
of pain

Then press an aluminium comb on to the fingertips as near as possible to the fingernails for thirty seconds:

1 On the left hand

2 On the right hand

Now massage the following pressure points for ten seconds each on the palm of your left hand:

1 The brain

2 The penial gland

3 The pituitary gland

4 The neck and cervicals

5 The spinal column

6 The main sinus

7 The eye

8 The eye sinus

9 The eye II

10 The eye sinus II

11 The ear

12 The ear sinus

13 The ear II

14 The ear sinus II

15 The ear nerves

16 The ear nerves II

17 The optical nerve

18 The optical nerve II

19 The eye III

20 The eye IV

21 The ear III

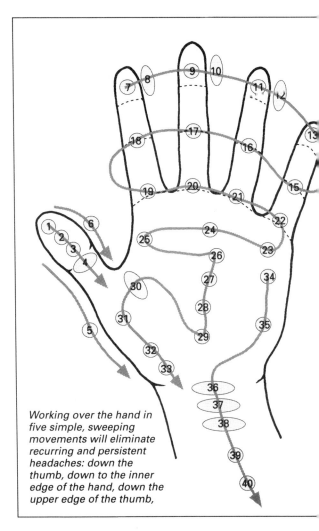

Working over the hand in five simple, sweeping movements will eliminate recurring and persistent headaches: down the thumb, down to the inner edge of the hand, down the upper edge of the thumb,

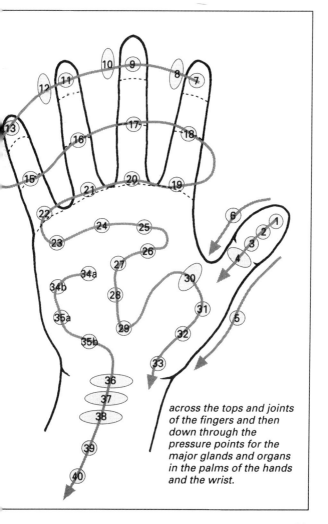

across the tops and joints of the fingers and then down through the pressure points for the major glands and organs in the palms of the hands and the wrist.

31

Now work on the right hand with the forefinger of the left hand. The pressure points on the right hand are the same as on the left except that pressure point 34 is here the gall bladder and liver rather than the spleen. The gall bladder is approximately a quarter of an inch to the right of the liver and approximately a quarter of an inch above it. Lastly, when you massage number 35, the descending colon on the left hand becomes the ascending colon on the right hand where it must be followed by the ileo-cecal pressure point which lies approximately a quarter of an inch below the kidney pressure point and half an inch to the left.

Now turn the left hand so that the palm is facing downwards and work on the following pressure points on the back of the left hand with your right hand; work on each pressure point for twenty seconds:

1 Between the nail and first joint of the thumb

2 In the small valley between the third and little finger

3 Across the back of the whole of the hand

4 Where the thumb joins the hand down to where the thumb joins the wrist

5 In the hollow where the hand joins the wrist

6 Six inches above the wrist

33

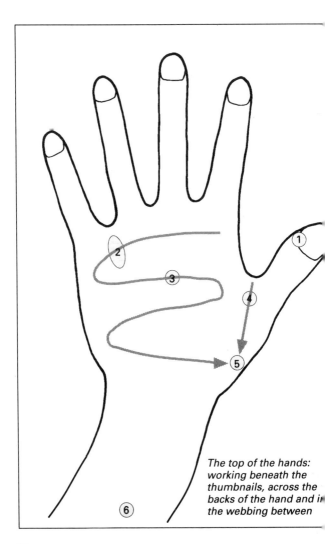

The top of the hands: working beneath the thumbnails, across the backs of the hand and in the webbing between

34

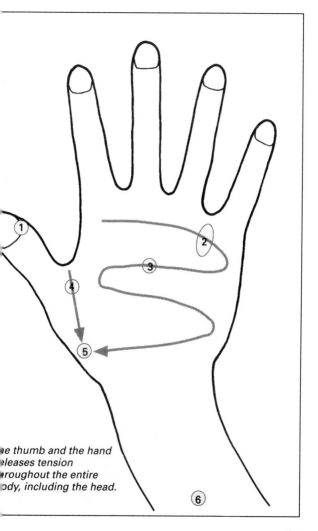

e thumb and the hand
eleases tension
roughout the entire
ody, including the head.

35

Now perform the same massage on the back of the right hand.

Turning your attention to the head, massage the following pressure points for thirty seconds each:

1 Where the back of the
  head joins the neck

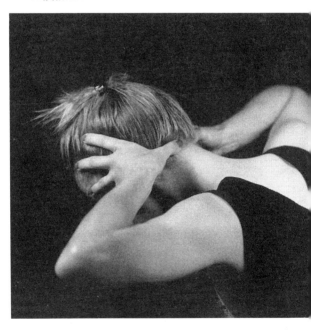

Working the point where the neck meets the head.

Working the highest point of the head

2 On the top of your
  head in the middle

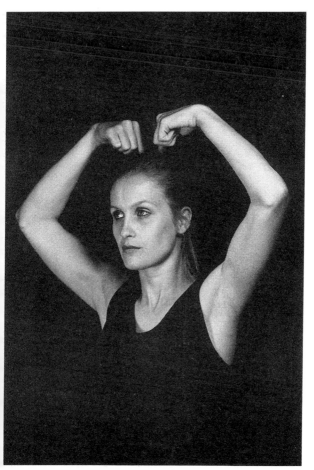

3 The temples

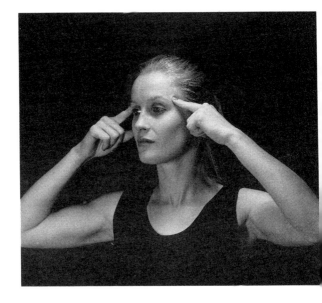

Massaging the temples.

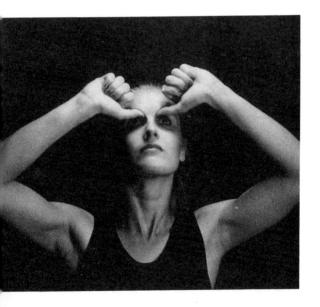

Massaging the bridge of bone underneath the eyebrows.

5 In the centre of the forehead

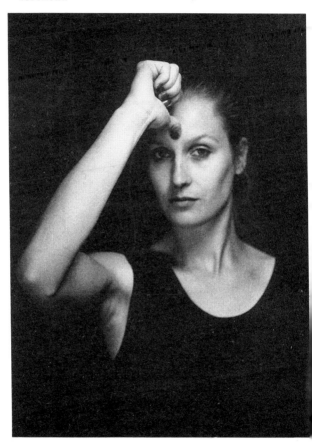

Massaging the pressure point for the pituitary gland in the middle of the forehead.

Now massage the following pressure points on the sole of your left foot for ten seconds:

1 The brain
2 The penial gland
3 The pituitary gland
4 The neck and cervicals
5 The main sinus
6 The eye sinus
7 The eye sinus II
8 The ear sinus
9 The ear sinus II
10 The ear reflex
11 The ear reflex II
12 The eye reflex
13 The eye reflex II
14 The spinal column
15 The lungs
16 The chest
17 The bronchials
18 The parathyroid and thyroid
19 The stomach
20 The pancreas
21 The thymus
22 The central nervous system
23 The spleen (on right

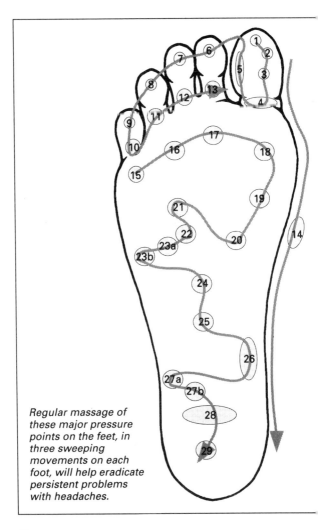

Regular massage of these major pressure points on the feet, in three sweeping movements on each foot, will help eradicate persistent problems with headaches.

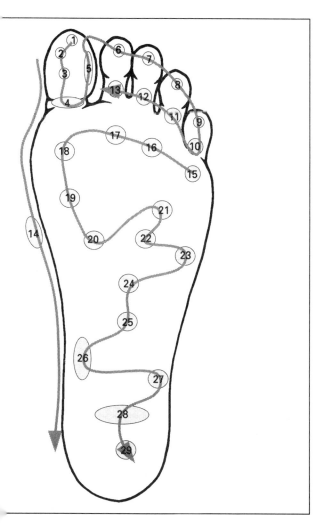

foot: 23a gall bladder,
23b liver)

24 The adrenal gland

25 The kidney

26 The bladder

27 The descending colon
(on right foot: 27a
ascending colon, 27b
ileo-cecal)

28 The sigmoid colon

29 The sciatic nerve

Now work on the sole of the right foot. The pressure points are the same as those on the left foot except that when you have massaged pressure point number 22, the central nervous system, you must move to massage the gall bladder pressure point which is approximately a quarter of an inch below the central nervous system and half an inch to the left, and from there you must move to the liver which is adjacent on the edge of the foot. Also, after massaging no.26 the bladder, the pressure point which follows is the ascending rather than the descending colon, and then you must massage the pressure point for the ileo-cecal which lies towards the bottom of the pressure point for the bladder and approximately one inch to the left.

Now put your left foot on the ground and work on the following pressure points on the top of this foot for twenty seconds each:

1 On the big toe between
the nail and the first
joint

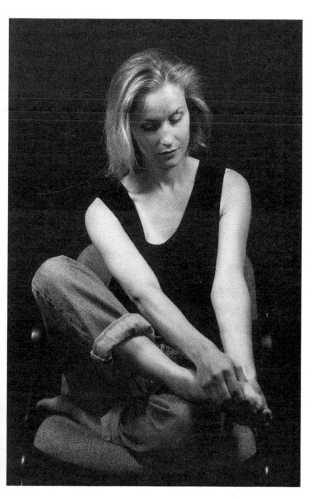

A comfortable position for massaging your own foot.

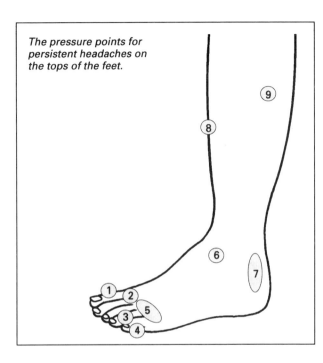

The pressure points for persistent headaches on the tops of the feet.

2 Where the big toe
  joins the foot

3 Behind the fourth
  toenail on the side
  closest to the little toe

4 Behind the outside
  corner of the nail on
  the little toe

5 Across the foot where

all the toes join the
foot

6 Where the foot joins or
meets the leg in line
with the separation
between the second
and third toes

7 In the hollow behind
the outer ankle

8 Place your thumb on
the bottom of your
kneecap and stretch
your hand as far down
your leg as possible;
where the middle
fingers reach on the
far side of the bone,
you will find a
pressure point

9 Place the heel of your
hand on the side of
your leg on the bottom
of your knee; where
the second finger
stretches to, you will
find the pressure point

Now perform the same exercises on the top of the right
foot.

Finally, perform the following relaxation exercise
which is an effective way of controlling the restless,
fragmented thinking and anxiety which is a big contribu-
tory factor to headaches.

You will need fifteen to twenty minutes when you know you will not be disturbed.

Make yourself comfortable by lying down on the floor and placing a telephone book under your head. Completely relax your toes, feet and ankles, your calves, knees and thighs, your stomach, chest, neck, throat, eyes, ears, scalp, shoulders, back, spine, arms, hands and fingers – make this a pleasant sensation.

Inhale a complete breath very slowly but steadily through the nostrils. Retain this breath for twenty seconds, then expel it as vigorously as possible in one breath through your mouth. Repeat six times.

Now, breathing through the nostrils, inhale steadily, filling first the lower part of the lung by pulling your diaphragm downwards. Then push forward the front wall of the abdomen, thus filling the middle part of the lungs. Then push out the lower ribs, breastbone and chest, and finally protrude the upper chest, thus filling the top of the lungs too.

Retain this breath for thirty seconds.

Exhale slowly keeping the chest in the same position, but drawing the abdomen inwards and lifting it upwards as the air leaves the lungs. Only when the air is entirely expelled must you relax the chest and abdomen.

The predominant feeling must be that of the pain leaving your body and your mind. The power flowing through you will make this a reality.

God bless you.

Joseph Corvo.